The Ultimate Dash Diet Recipe Book

Easy And Tasty Dash Diet Recipes To Lose Weight

Peter Haley

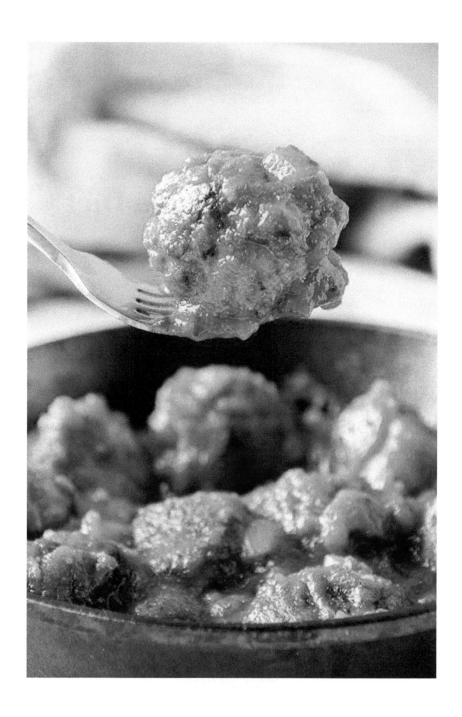

Table of contents

Berry Soufflé

Prep time: 15 mins

Servings: 2

Cooking: 15 mins

Ingredients:

- 2 tbsp sugar
- ½ cup water
- 3 oz. rinsed berries
- 3 egg whites

Directions:

1. Combine the berries sugar and water in a saucepan and boil until thick.
2. Using an electric beater beat the egg whites until foamy.
3. Constantly stirring, combine the berry mixture with egg whites.
4. Pour the soufflé mixture into a mold.
5. Bake at 390°F for 15 mins.

6. Serve immediately, sprinkled with confectioners' sugar if desired.

Nutrition:

- Calories 79
- Fat 0.4 g
- Carbs 28.6 g
- Protein 8.3 g

Stuffed Turnips

Prep time: 5 mins

Servings: 4

Cooking: 1 hour

Ingredients:

- 2 peeled and grated carrots
- 2 tbsp Olive oil
- 2 tbsp Honey
- 4 rinsed turnips.
- 2 peeled and grated apples

Directions:

1. Preheat the oven to 400°F.
2. Mix grated carrots with grated apples in honey.
3. Boil the turnips until half-done.
4. When the turnips are cool enough to handle, cut off the tops and scoop out some of the flesh.

5. Rub the turnips inside with olive oil and fill with vegetable stuffing.
6. Bake for 1 hr.

Nutrition:

- Calories 197
- Fat 7.3 g
- Carbs 8 g
- Protein 4 g

Roasted Asparagus

Prep time: 1 hour

Servings: 2

Ingredients:

- Black pepper
- 1 tsp. olive oil
- 2 cup quartered mushrooms
- Zest of 1 lemon
- 1 lb. sliced asparagus
- 2 tbsp Balsamic vinegar

Directions:

1. In a bowl combine all ingredients: until well coated.
2. Place into the fridge for 1 hour to marinate.
3. Broil the asparagus mixture under high heat until lightly browned.

Nutrition:

- Calories 143
- Fat 7.6 g
- Carbs 3.9 g
- Protein 22 g

Brussels Sprouts with Walnuts

Prep time: 10 mins

Servings: 4

Ingredients:

- ½ cup fresh shaved parmesan
- 1 tsp. thyme
- 2 tbsp olive oil
- 1 tsp. black pepper
- ½ cup chopped walnuts
- ½ cup diced red onion
- 4 cup shaved Brussels sprouts

Directions:

1. Heat the olive oil in a skillet over medium heat. Add the onions and sauté until tender, approximately 2-3 mins.
2. Add the Brussels sprouts and cook for 5 mins. Season with thyme and black pepper.
3. Remove from heat and stir in the walnuts.

4. Garnish with fresh Parmesan for serving.

Nutrition:

- Calories 173.0
- Fat 12.8 g
- Carbs 10.0 g
- Protein 5.7 g

Grilled Pesto Shrimps

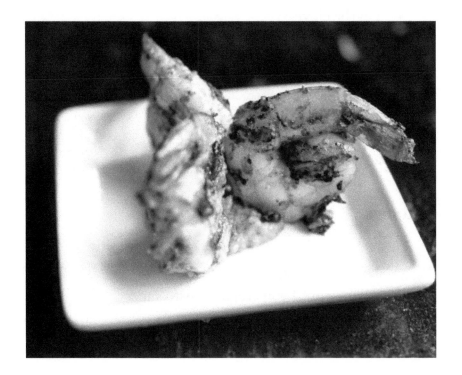

Prep time: 10 mins

Servings: 2

Cooking: 3/4 mins

Ingredients:

- 1 garlic clove
- ¼ kg. peeled and deveined large shrimp
- ½ cup chopped basil
- Skewers
- 2 tbsp olive oil
- 2 tbsp parmesan cheese

Directions:

1. Place the fresh basil, garlic, cheese, salt and pepper in a food processor and pulse. Gradually add the oil to the mixture until you create a pesto sauce.
2. Place the shrimps in a bowl and pour over the pesto sauce. Toss gently and let it marinate in t fridge for at least an hour.
3. When you're ready to cook, pre-heat your grill to medium-low heat.
4. Thread the shrimps into the skewers and cook on the grill for about 3-4 mins on each side.
5. Serve warm with a bowl of yogurt and fresh fruits.

Nutrition:

- Calories 219.7
- Fat 7.8 g
- Carbs 22.2 g
- Protein 15.1 g

Rosemary Potato Shells

Prep time: 5 mins

Servings: 2

Cooking: 1 hour

Ingredients:

- Butter-flavored cooking spray
- 2 medium russet potatoes
- 1/8 tsp. freshly ground black pepper
- 1 tbsp minced fresh rosemary

Directions:

1. Switch on the oven and set it to 375 º F to preheat.
2. Pierce the mashed potatoes with a fork and place them in a baking sheet.
3. Bake for 1 hour until crispy.
4. Allow the potatoes to cool for handling then cut them in half.
5. Scoop out the pulp leaving the 1/8-inch-thick shell.

6. Brush the shells with melted butter and season with pepper and rosemary.
7. Bake for another 5 mins.
8. Serve.

Nutrition:

- Calories 167
- Fat 0 g
- Carbs 27 g
- Protein 7.6 g

Basil Tomato Crostini

Prep time: 10 mins

Servings: 4

Cooking: 30 mins

Ingredients:

- ¼ cup minced fresh basil
- ¼ lb. sliced and toasted bread
- 4 chopped plum tomatoes
- 2 tsps. olive oil
- Freshly ground pepper
- 1 minced garlic clove

Directions:

1. Toss tomatoes with oil, garlic, pepper, and basil in a bowl.
2. Cover and allow them sit for 30 mins.
3. Top the toasts with this mixture.
4. Serve.

Nutrition:

- Calories 104
- Fat 3.5 g
- Carbs 15 g
- Protein 3 g

Cranberry Spritzer

Prep time: 10 mins

Servings: 4

Ingredients:

- 1 cup raspberry sherbet
- 1-quart sugar-free cranberry juice
- ¼ cup sugar
- 10 lemon wedges
- ½ cup fresh lemon juice
- 1-quart carbonated water

Directions:

1. Refrigerate carbonated water, lemon juice, and cranberry juice until cold.
2. Mix cranberry juice with sugar, sherbet, lemon juice, and carbonated water.
3. Garnish with a lemon wedge.
4. Serve.

Nutrition:

- Calories 50
- Fat 0 g
- Carbs 15.1 g
- Protein 1.2 g

Penne with Broccoli

Prep time: 5 mins

Servings: 2

Cooking: 10 mins

Ingredients:

- 3 minced garlic cloves
- 2 tbsp grated parmesan cheese
- Pepper.
- 1/3 lb. Penne pasta
- 2 cup broccoli florets
- 2 tsps. olive oil

Directions:

1. Fill a large saucepan with water and bring to a boil. Following the instructions on the package add the pasta and cook until al dente.

2. In a separate pot add 1 inch water and bring to boil. Put the broccoli florets into a steamer basket and steam for 10 mins.
3. In a large bowl combine the cooked pasta with broccoli. Toss with garlic, olive oil, Parmesan cheese, and black pepper.

Nutrition:

- Calories 46.2
- Fat 14.9 g
- Carbs 25 g
- Protein 14 g

White Sponge Cake

Prep time: 15 mins

Servings: 4

Cooking: 20 mins

Ingredients:

- 1 tbsp sugar
- 1 tbsp flour
- 2 egg whites

Directions:

1. Using an electric mixer beat the egg whites until foamy.
2. Slowly add sugar, continuing to whisk.
3. Slowly add the flour, constantly stirring.
4. Pour the mixture into a silicone mold.
5. Bake at 400F for 20 min. Check for doneness with a toothpick.

Nutrition:

- Calories 23
- Fat 0.1 g
- Carbs 36.4 g
- Protein 4.6 g

Pan Seared Acorn Squash and Pecans

Prep time: 5 mins

Servings: 6

Cooking: 13 mins

Ingredients:

- 1 tsp. chopped rosemary
- 1 cup sliced sweet yellow onion
- 2 tbsp vegetable oil
- 4 cup cubed acorn squash
- 1 tbsp honey
- 1 cup chopped pecans

Directions:

1. Add the vegetable oil to a sauté pan over medium high heat.
2. Add the onion and sauté until tender, 2-3 mins.
3. Add the acorn squash, tossing gently for 5-7 mins.

4. Add the honey, pecans, and rosemary. Stir to coat and cook an additional 3 mins.
5. Serve warm.

Nutrition:

- Calories 222.3
- Fat 17.6 g
- Carbs 17.4 g
- Protein 2.7 g

Squash Pancakes

Prep time: 10 mins

Servings: 4

Cooking: 20-30 mins

Ingredients:

- 2 beaten eggs
- Sour cream
- 2 peeled, deseeded and grated medium summer squashes
- 1 tbsp flour

Directions:

1. Drain the liquid from the grated squashes.
2. Add eggs, flour and season with salt. Mix well. Form this mixture into pancakes.
3. Line a baking sheet with parchment paper and scoop the pancakes onto it.
4. Bake in the oven at 400F for 20-30 mins.

5. Serve with sour cream.

Nutrition:

- Calories 31
- Fat 0.4 g
- Carbs 12.7 g
- Protein 5.8 g

Apples Stuffed with Quark

Prep time: 5 mins

Servings: 4

Cooking: 20 mins

Ingredients:

- 8 oz. cottage cheese
- 1 tsp. confectioners' sugar
- 2 tbsp Sugar
- 4 cored apples
- 1 whisked egg
- 1 tbsp raisins

Directions:

1. Combine the quark with egg, sugar and raisins. Mix well.
2. Scrape out the some of the apples' flesh and fill with quark mixture.
3. Place on a baking sheet and bake at 400F for 20 mins.

Nutrition:

- Calories 189
- Fat 0.6 g
- Carbs 9 g
- Protein 12 g

Meringue Cookies

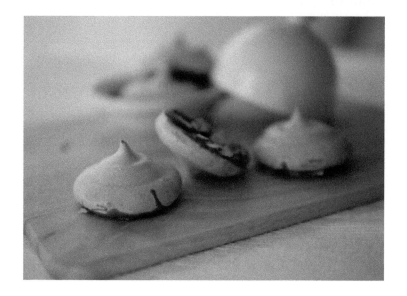

Prep time: 5 mins

Servings: 4

Cooking: 15 mins

Ingredients:

- 2 tbsp Sugar
- 3 beaten egg whites

Directions:

1. Using a blender beat the cooled egg whites on high.
2. Constantly blending add sugar little by little.
3. Line a baking sheet with parchment paper. Using an icing bag, squeeze our portions of the egg mixture unto the parchment paper.
4. Place into a preheated to 155°F oven for 15 min.

Nutrition:

- Calories 35
- Fat 0 g
- Carbs 6 g
- Protein 0.4 g

Rose Hip Jelly

Prep time: 7 hours

Servings: 2

Ingredients:

- 2 cup water
- 1 tsp. gelatin
- 2 tbsp Sugar
- 2 tbsp Rinsed and crushed rose-hip berries
- 2 lemon slices

Directions:

1. Bring the 2 cups water to a boil, add the crushed rose hips and boil for 5 mins
2. Leave the hips in the liquid to infuse for 6 hours. Then strain the infusion through a sieve, retaining the liquid.
3. Dissolve sugar in ½ cup of rose-hip water and bring to boil. Add the remaining rose-hip water and lemon slices.
4. Soak the gelatin in cool water for 25-30 mins.

5. Add the gelatin to the rose-hip extract and bring to a boil. Take it from the heat immediately and pour into molds or jars

6. Place in the fridge to cool and thicken.

Nutrition:

- Calories 45
- Fat 0 g
- Carbs 11 g
- Protein 0 g

Easy Broccoli and Pasta

Prep time: 10 mins

Servings: 3

Ingredients:

- 3 chopped garlic cloves
- 6 oz. uncooked whole-wheat pasta
- Ground pepper
- 3 cup roughly chopped broccoli florets
- 1 tbsp olive oil
- 2 tbsp Grated Romano cheese

Directions:

1. Cook the penne in a pot according to the package instructions. Add the florets to cook with the pasta.
2. Before draining, take ¼ cup of the pasta water and set aside.
3. Place the pot back to the stove and heat the olive oil over high heat. Sauté the garlic for about a minute.
4. Reduce the heat and then add the pasta and broccoli to the pot. Stir well.

5. Add the Romano and ¼ cup of the pasta water. Mix well. Season with pepper.

Nutrition:

- Calories 419.8
- Fat 12.9 g
- Carbs 52 g
- Protein 32.2 g

Hearty Chia And Blackberry Pudding

Prep time: 45 mins

Servings: 2

Ingredients:

- ¼ cup chia seeds
- ½ cup blackberries, fresh
- 1 tsp liquid sweetener
- 1 cup coconut almond milk, full fat and unsweetened
- 1 tsp vanilla extract

Directions:

1. Take the vanilla, liquid sweetener and coconut almond milk and add to blender
2. Process until thick
3. Add in blackberries and process until smooth
4. Divide the mixture between cups and chill for 30 mins

Nutrition:

- Calories 314.8
- Fat 25.0 g
- Carbs 22.1 g
- Protein 4.5 g

Special Cocoa Brownies

Prep time: 15 mins

Servings: 12

Cooking time: 25 mins

Ingredients:

- 2 tbsps grass-fed almond butter
- 1 whole egg
- 2 tsps vanilla extract
- ¼ tsp baking powder
- 1/3 cup heavy cream
- 3/4 cup almond butter
- ¼ cocoa powder
- A pinch of sunflower seeds

Directions:

1. Break the eggs and whisk until smooth
2. Add in all the wet ingredients: and mix well

3. Make the batter by mixing all the dry ingredients: and sifting them into the wet ingredients:
4. Pour into a greased baking pan Bake for 25 mins at 350 degrees F or until a toothpick inserted in the middle comes out clean

Nutrition:

- Calories 355.8
- Fat 25.0 g
- Carbs 22.1 g
- Protein 4.5 g

Gentle Blackberry Crumble

Prep time: 10 mins

Servings: 4

Cooking time: 45 mins

Ingredients:

- ½ a cup of coconut flour
- ½ a cup of banana, peeled and mashed
- 6 tbsp of water
- 3 cups of fresh blackberries
- ½ a cup of arrowroot flour
- 1 and a ½ tsp of baking soda
- 4 tbsp of almond butter, melted
- 1 tbsp of fresh lemon juice

Directions:

1. Pre-heat your oven to 300 degrees F
2. Take a baking dish and grease it lightly

3. Take a bowl and mix all of the ingredients: except blackberries, mix well
4. Place blackberries in the bottom of your baking dish and top with flour
5. Bake for 40 mins

Nutrition:

- Calories 325.8
- Fat 20.0 g
- Carbs 22.1 g
- Protein 5.5 g

Nutmeg Nougats

Prep time: 10 mins

Servings: 12

Cooking time: 5 mins +30mins

Freeze Time: 30 mins

Ingredients:

- 1 cup coconut, shredded
- 1 cup low-fat cream
- 1 cup cashew almond butter
- ½ tsp ground nutmeg

Directions:

1. Melt the cashew almond butter over a double boiler
2. Stir in nutmeg and dairy cream
3. Remove from the heat
4. Allow to cool down a little

5. Keep in the refrigerator for at least 30 mins
6. Take out from the fridge and make small balls
7. Coat with shredded coconut
8. Let it cool for 2 hours and then serve

Nutrition:

- Calories 334
- Fat 28.0 g
- Carbs 20.1 g
- Protein 4.5 g

Apple And Almond Muffins

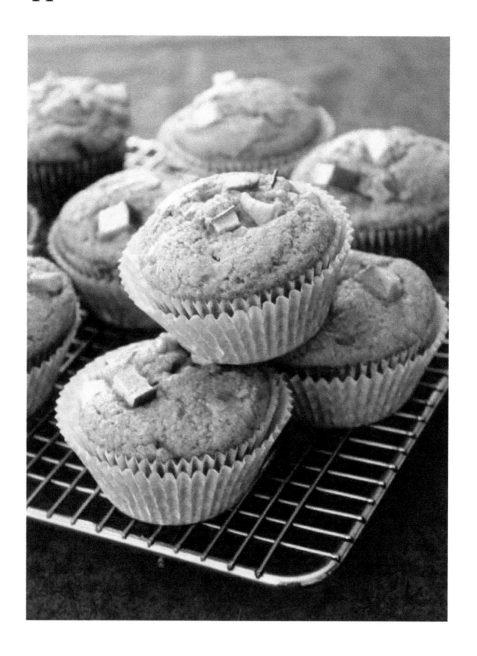

Prep time: 10 mins

Servings: 6

Cooking time: 20 mins

Ingredients:

- 6 oz ground almonds
- 1 tsp cinnamon
- ½ tsp baking powder
- 1 pinch sunflower seeds
- 1 whole egg
- 1 tsp apple cider vinegar
- 2 tbsps Erythritol
- 1/3 cup apple sauce

Directions:

1. Pre-heat your oven to 350° F
2. Line muffin tin with paper muffin cups, keep them on the side
3. Mix in almonds, cinnamon, baking powder, sunflower seeds and keep it on the side

4. Take another bowl and beat in eggs, apple cider vinegar, apple sauce, Erythritol
5. Add the mix to dry ingredients: and mix well until you have a smooth batter
6. Pour batter into tin and bake for 20 mins
7. Once done, let them cool

Nutrition:

- Calories 314
- Fat 21.0 g
- Carbs 18.1 g
- Protein 6.5 g

Sweet Potatoes and Apples Mix

Prep time: 10 mins

Servings: 1

Ingredients:

- 1 tbsp low-fat butter
- ½ lb. cored and chopped apples
- 2 tbsp water
- 2 lbs. sweet potatoes

Directions:

1. Arrange the potatoes around the lined baking sheet, bake inside oven at 400 º F for an hour, peel them and mash them in the meat processor.
2. Put apples in the very pot, add the river, bring using a boil over medium heat, reduce temperature, and cook for ten mins.
3. Transfer to your bowl, add mashed potatoes, stir well and serve every day.
4. Enjoy!

Nutrition:

- Calories 140
- Fat 1 g
- Carbs 8 g
- Protein 6 g

Sautéed Bananas with Orange Sauce

Prep time: 5 mins

Servings: 4

Ingredients:

- ¼ cup frozen pure orange juice concentrate
- 2 tbsp margarine
- ¼ cup sliced almonds
- 1 tsp. orange zest
- 1 tsp. fresh grated ginger
- 4 firm, sliced ripe bananas
- 1 tsp. cinnamon

Directions:

1. Melt the margarine over medium heat in a large skillet, until it bubbles but before it begins to brown.
2. Add the cinnamon, ginger, and orange zest. Cook, while stirring, for 1 minute before adding the orange juice concentrate. Cook, while stirring until an even sauce has formed.

3. Add the bananas and cook, stirring carefully for 1-2 mins, or until warmed and evenly coated with the sauce.
4. Serve warm with sliced almonds.

Nutrition:

- Calories 164.3
- Fat 9.0 g
- Carbs 21.4 g
- Protein 2.3 g

Caramelized Apricot

Prep time: 10 mins

Servings: 6

Ingredients:

- ¼ cup white sugar
- 2 tsps. lemon juice
- ½ tsp. thyme
- 3 cup sliced apricots
- 1 tbsp brown sugar
- 1 cup part skim ricotta cheese
- 1 tsp. lemon zest

Directions:

1. Preheat the broiler of your oven.
2. Place the apricots in a bowl and toss with the lemon juice.
3. In another bowl, combine the ricotta cheese, thyme, and lemon zest. Mix well.

4. Spread a layer of the ricotta mixture into the bottoms of 6 large baking ramekins.
5. Spoon the apricots over the top of the ricotta cheese in each.
6. Combine the white sugar and brown sugar. Sprinkle evenly over the apricots, avoiding large clumps of sugar as much as possible.
7. Place the ramekins under the broiler for approximately 5 mins, or until caramelized.
8. Serve warm.

Nutrition:

- Calories 133.6
- Fat 3.6 g
- Carbs 21.6 g
- Protein 5.8 g

Rhubarb Pie

Prep time: 10 mins

Servings: 12

Ingredients:

- 4 cup chopped rhubarb
- 8 oz. low-fat cream cheese
- 1 cup melted low-fat butter
- 1 ¼ cup coconut sugar
- 2 cup whole wheat flour
- 1 cup chopped pecans
- 1 cup sliced strawberries

Directions:

1. In a bowl, combine the flour while using the butter, pecans and ¼ cup sugar and stir well.
2. Transfer this for some pie pan, press well in for the pan, introduce inside the oven and bake at 350 º F for 20 mins.

3. In a pan, combine the strawberries with all the current rhubarb, cream cheese and 1 cup sugar, stir well and cook over medium heat for 4 mins.
4. Spread this inside the pie crust whilst inside fridge for the couple hours before slicing and serving.

Nutrition:

- Calories 162
- Fat 5 g
- Carbs 15 g
- Protein 6 g

Berry Bars

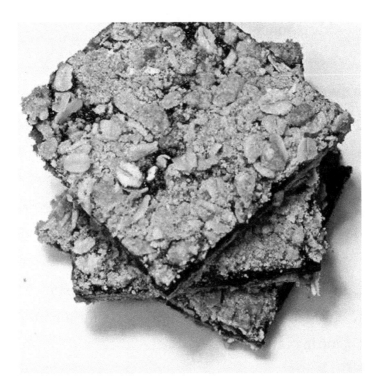

Prep time: 10 mins

Servings: 18

Ingredients:

- 1 cup natural peanut butter
- ¼ cup chopped dried blueberries

- 3 cup oatmeal
- ¼ cup chopped dried cranberries
- 3 tbsp honey

Directions:

1. Line a baking pan with wax paper or parchment paper.
2. Microwave the peanut butter for 10-15 seconds, just until it softens and begins to liquefy.
3. Combine the oatmeal, peanut butter, honey, cranberries, and blueberries together in a bowl and mix until blended.
4. Spread the mixture out evenly into the pan.
5. Place in the refrigerator and let set for 2 hours before cutting into squares.

Nutrition:

- Calories 145.0
- Fat 6.4 g
- Carbs 17.9 g
- Protein 4.4 g

Chocolate Avocado Pudding

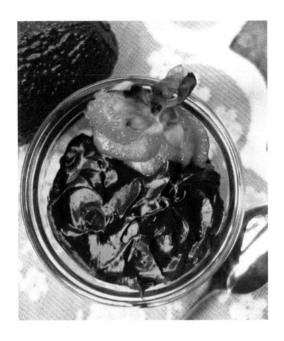

Prep time: 30 mins

Servings: 2

Ingredients:

- 1 avocado, chunked
- 1 tbsp natural sweetener such as stevia
- 2 oz cream cheese, at room temp
- ¼ tsp vanilla extract

61

- 4 tbsps cocoa powder, unsweetened

Directions:

1. Blend listed ingredients: in blender until smooth
2. Divide the mix between dessert bowls, chill for 30 mins

Nutrition:

- Calories 284
- Fat 18.0 g
- Carbs 20.1 g
- Protein 5.5 g

Ginger Peach Pie

Prep time: 10 mins

Servings: 10

Ingredients:

- 5 cup diced peaches
- ½ cup sugar
- 2 refrigerated whole wheat pie crust doughs
- 1 tsp. cinnamon
- ½ cup orange juice
- ¼ cup chopped candied ginger
- ½ cup cornstarch

Directions:

1. Preheat the oven to 425°F.
2. Place one of the pie crusts in a standard size pie dish. Spread some coffee beans or dried beans in the bottom of the pie crust to use as a weight. Place the dish in the oven and bake for 10-15 mins, or until lightly golden. Remove from the oven and let cool.

3. Combine the peaches, candied ginger, and cinnamon in a bowl. Toss to mix.
4. Combine the sugar, cornstarch, and orange juice in a saucepan and heat over medium until syrup begins to thicken.
5. Pour the syrup over the peaches and toss to coat.
6. Spread the peaches in the pie crust and top with the remaining crust. Crimp along the edges and cut several small slits in the top.
7. Place in the oven and bake for 25-30 mins, or until golden brown.
8. Let set before slicing.

Nutrition:

- Calories 289.0
- Fat 13.1 g
- Carbs 41.6 g
- Protein 3.9 g

Pomegranate Mix

Prep time: 10 mins

Servings: 2

Ingredients:

- Single pomegranate seeds
- 2 cup pomegranate juice
- 1 cup steel cut oats

Directions:

In a bit pot, combine the pomegranate juice with pomegranate seeds and oats, toss, cook over medium heat for 5 mins, divide into bowls and serve cold.

Nutrition:

- Calories 172
- Fat 4 g
- Carbs 10 g
- Protein 5 g

Oriental Rice

Prep time: 5 mins

Servings: 6

Cooking: 13 mins

Ingredients:

- 1-1/2 cups water
- 1 cup chicken stock or broth, skim fat from top
- 1-1/3 cups uncooked long-grain white rice
- 2 tsps vegetable oil
- 2 tbsps finely chopped onion
- 2 T finely chopped green pepper
- 1/2 cup chopped pecans
- 1/4 tsp ground sage
- 1 cup finely chopped celery
- 1/2 cup sliced water chestnuts
- 1/4 tsp nutmeg

Directions:

1. Bring water and stock to a boil in medium-size saucepan.
2. Add rice and stir. Cover and simmer 20 mins.
3. Remove pan from heat. Let stand, covered, 5 mins or until all liquid is absorbed. Reserve.
4. Heat oil in large nonstick skillet.
5. Sauté onion and celery over moderate heat 3 mins. Stir in remaining ingredients: including reserved cooked rice. Fluff with fork before serving.

Nutrition:

- Calories 139
- Total Fat 5 g
- Saturated Fat less

Parmesan Rice and Pasta Pilaf

Prep time: 5 mins

Servings: 6

Cooking: 13 mins

Ingredients:

- 2 tbsps olive oil
- 1/2 cup finely broken vermicelli, uncooked
- 2 tbsps diced onion
- 1 cup long-grain white rice, uncooked
- 1-1/4 cups hot chicken stock
- 1-1/4 cups hot water
- 1/4 tsp ground white pepper
- 1 bay leaf
- 2 tbsps grated parmesan cheese

Directions:

1. In a large skillet, heat oil. Sauté vermicelli and onion until golden brown, about 2 to 4 mins over medium-high heat. Drain off oil.
2. Add rice, stock, water, pepper, and bay leaf. Cover and simmer 15-20 mins. Fluff with fork. Cover and let stand 5-20 mins. Remove bay leaf.
3. Sprinkle with cheese and serve immediately.

Nutrition:

- Calories 172

- Fat 6 g

Roasted Carrots

Prep time: 15 mins

Servings: 4

Cooking: 30 mins

Ingredients:

- 2 lbs. peeled and halved carrots
- 2 tbsp olive oil
- Flat leaf parsley
- 1 tbsp raw honey

Directions:

1. Preheat the oven to 400F.
2. Peel the carrots, cutting off the stems, and then cut the carrots in half creating a piece with a wide and narrow half.
3. Halve each carrot in half again lengthwise.

4. Place all the cut carrots into a bowl and add the olive oil, salt, pepper, and raw honey. Toss the carrots well to coat.

5. Spread the carrots evenly onto a baking sheet lined with aluminum foil, making sure they are all in a single layer.

6. Bake the carrots for 30 mins, and then remove from oven to cool.

7. Garnish with fresh flat leaf parsley, if desired.

Nutrition:

- Calories 109
- Fat 5.8 g
- Carbs 14 g
- Protein 1.4 g

Turkey and Cheese Sandwich

Prep time: 10 mins

Servings: 2

Cooking: 5 mins

Ingredients:

- 2 tsps. Dijon mustard
- ½ cup thinly sliced cucumber
- 2 whole-grain bread slices
- 2 low-sodium smoked turkey slices
- Pepper.
- ¼ cup shredded low-fat mozzarella

Directions:

1. Spread the mustard on each of the slices.
2. Lay the smoked turkey slice and then the cucumber slices on top of the bread. Sprinkle with the mozzarella and season with pepper.
3. Toaster to melt the cheese for about 3 mins.
4. Serve while warm.

Nutrition:

- Calories 380
- Fat 13.5 g
- Carbs 40 g
- Protein 25 g

Crunchy Mashed Sweet Potatoes

Prep time: 5 mins

Servings: 4

Cooking: 10 mins

Ingredients:

- ¼ tsp. nutmeg
- 1 cup water
- 2 lbs. Sliced garnet sweet potatoes
- Sea flavored vinegar
- 2 tbsp Maple syrup
- 3 tbsp Vegan butter

Directions:

1. Peel the sweet potatoes and cut up into 1 inch chunks
2. Pour 1 cup of water to the pot and add steamer basket
3. Add sweet potato chunks in the basket
4. Lock up the lid and cook on HIGH pressure for 8 mins
5. Quick release the pressure

6. Open the lid and place the cooked sweet potatoes to the bowl
7. Use a masher to mash the potatoes
8. Add ¼ tsp of nutmeg, 2-3 tbsp of unflavored vinegar butter, 2 tbsp of maple syrup
9. Mash and mix
10. Season with flavored vinegar

Nutrition:

- Calories 249
- Fat 8 g
- Carbs 37 g
- Protein 7 g

Special Roast Potatoes

Prep time: 5 mins

Servings: 4

Cooking: 17 mins

Ingredients:

- Pepper
- 2 lbs. baby potatoes
- 3 skinned out garlic clove
- ½ cup stock
- 5 tbsp Olive oil
- 1 rosemary sprig

Directions:

1. Set your pot to Sauté mode and add oil
2. Once it is heated up, add in the garlic, rosemary and potatoes
3. Sauté the potatoes for 10 mins and brown them

4. Take a sharp knife and cut a small piece in the middle of your potatoes and pour the stock

5. Lock up the lid and cook on HIGH pressure for 7 mins

6. Once done, wait for 10 mins and release the pressure naturally

7. Add garlic cloves and peel the potatoes skin

8. Sprinkle a bit of pepper and enjoy!

Nutrition:

- Calories 42
- Fat 1.3 g
- Carbs 7.3 g
- Protein 0.8 g

Crazy Eggs

Prep time: 5 mins

Servings: 6

Cooking: 10 mins

Ingredients:

- Guacamole
- Furikake
- Mayonnaise
- 8 large eggs
- 1 cup water
- Sliced radishes

Directions:

1. Add 1 cup of water to your Instant Pot
2. Place the steamer insert in your pot
3. Arrange the eggs on top of the insert
4. Lock up the lid and cook for about 6 mins at HIGH pressure

5. Allow the pressure to release naturally

6. Transfer the eggs to an ice bath and peel the skin

7. Cut the eggs in half and garnish them with dressings of Guacamole, sliced up radishes, Mayonnaise, Furikake, Sliced up Parmesan etcup!

Nutrition:

- Calories 137
- Fat 10 g
- Carbs 1 g
- Protein 11 g

Potato, Onions and Bell Peppers

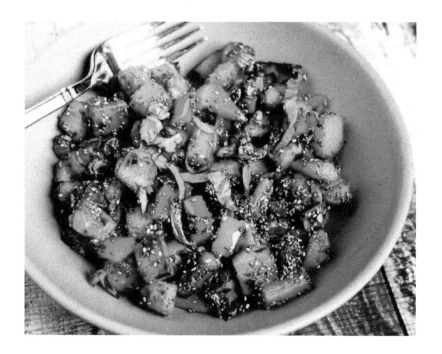

Prep time: 20 mins

Servings: 4

Cooking: 20 mins

Ingredients:

- 2 cups water
- 2 large russet potatoes, cleaned and cut in half
- 1 tbsp vegetable oil
- 1/2 cup chopped onion
- 1/2 cup chopped green and red bell pepper
- 1/2 cup no salt added canned corn or frozen corn, thawed
- 1/2 cup chopped tomato
- 1/2 tsp oregano
- 1/4 cup crumbled reduced fat Monterey Jack cheese

Directions:

1. Bring water to a boil in a large pan. Add potatoes and cook until crisp-tender, about 15 mins. Drain well and cut into bite-size pieces.
2. Heat oil in a large skillet. Sauté onion until golden brown and soft. Add potatoes and bell pepper to skillet and cook over medium-high heat, stirring frequently, until golden brown.
3. Stir in corn, tomato, oregano, salt, and ground black pepper. Top with cheese and serve.

Nutrition:

- Calories 217
- Carbs 39 g
- Protein 6 g
- Fat 5 g

Green Pea Purée

Prep time: 20 mins

Servings: 2

Ingredients:

- 2 boiled sliced carrots
- ¼ cup 20% fat sour cream
- Pepper.
- 2 cup green peas

Directions:

1. Boil the carrots and the peas.
2. Using a blender purée the vegetables. Season with salt and pepper. Top with sour cream.

Nutrition:

- Calories 101
- Fat 2.1 g
- Carbs 14 g
- Protein 7 g

Green Beans with Nuts

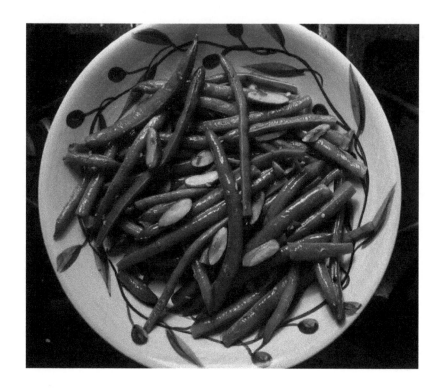

Prep time: 20 mins

Servings: 2

Cooking: 8 mins

Ingredients:

- 3 minced garlic cloves
- 1 tbsp olive oil
- ½ cup chopped walnuts
- 2 cup sliced green beans

Directions:

1. Boil the beans in salted water until tender.
2. Place the beans, garlic and walnuts in a preheated pan and cook for about 5-7 mins on the stove.

Nutrition:

- Calories 285
- Fat 24.1 g
- Carbs 7.1 g
- Protein 10 g

Beets Stewed with Apples

Prep time: 1 hour

Servings: 2

Cooking: 30 mins

Ingredients:

- 2 tbsp Tomato paste
- 1 tbsp Olive oil
- 1 cup water
- 2 peeled, cored and sliced apples
- 3 peeled, boiled and grated beets
- 2 tbsp Sour cream

Directions:

1. Boil the beets until half-done
2. In a deep pan preheated with olive oil cook the grated beets for 15 mins.
3. Add the sliced apples, tomato paste, sour cream and 1 cup water. Stew for 30 mins covered.

Nutrition:

- Calories 346
- Fat 7.7 g
- Carbs 26.8 g
- Protein 2 g

Cabbage Quiche

Prep time: 30 mins

Servings: 4

Ingredients:

- 2 beaten eggs
- 2 tbsp Sour cream
- 2 tsps. Semolina
- Fresh parsley
- ½ shredded white cabbage head
- 2 tbsp milk

Directions:

1. In a saucepan stew the shredded cabbage with milk until soft and done.
2. Sprinkle the semolina over the cabbage, constantly stirring, and cook for 10 mins more.
3. Remove from the heat, let cool and stir in the beaten eggs. Season with salt.
4. Arrange the cabbage mixture in a baking dish, coat with sour cream and bake at 400F for 20 mins.

5. Serve with sour cream and fresh parsley leaves.

Nutrition:

- Calories 93
- Fat 0.5 g
- Carbs 27.8 g
- Protein 19.4 g

Baked Tomatoes

Prep time: 5 mins

Servings: 2

Cooking: 10 mins

Ingredients:

- 2 minced garlic cloves
- 2 tbsp Olive oil
- 2 sliced large tomatoes
- 2 tbsp Minced basil
- 1 minced rosemary sprig

Directions:

1. Brush a baking sheet with olive oil.
2. Arrange the tomato slices on the baking sheet. Sprinkle with garlic, basil and rosemary. Brush with olive oil.
3. Bake in a preheated 350°F oven for 5-10 mins.

Nutrition:

- Calories 161
- Fat 14.5 g
- Carbs 2 g
- Protein 0.4 g

Cabbage Rolls with Dried Apricots

Prep time: 30 mins

Servings: 4

Cooking: 40 mins

Ingredients:

- 4 tbsp Rinsed and chopped dried apricots,
- 2 peeled, cored and grated apples
- 1/3 tsp. cinnamon
- 1 boiled cabbage head
- 2 tbsp Rinsed raisins
- 1 tbsp sugar

Directions:

1. Combine the grated apples, raisins, dried apricots, sugar and cinnamon.
2. Prepare the cabbage leaves: place the head of cabbage into water and bring to a boil. As the cabbage softens

take it out, remove the outer leaves and carefully peel the leaves off one by one.

3. Spread the leaves out on paper towels and fill with apricot stuffing. Roll them up.

4. Place the rolls into preheated to 400°F oven for 40 mins.

Nutrition:

- Calories 175
- Fat 0.4 g
- Carbs 16.6 g
- Protein 10.8 g

Herbed Green Beans

Prep time: 5 mins

Servings: 4

Cooking: 8 mins

Ingredients:

- ½ cup chopped fresh mint
- 2 minced garlic cloves
- 1 tsp. lemon zest
- 4 cup trimmed green beans
- 1 tbsp olive oil
- 1 tsp. coarse ground black pepper
- ½ cup chopped fresh parsley

Directions:

1. Heat the olive oil in a large sauté pan over medium heat. Add the green beans and garlic
2. Sauté until the green beans are crisp tender, approximately 5-6 mins.

3. Add the mint, parsley, lemon zest, and black pepper. Toss to coat.

Nutrition:

- Calories 66.2
- Fat 3.5 g
- Carbs 8.3 g
- Protein 2.1 g

Chickpea Meatballs

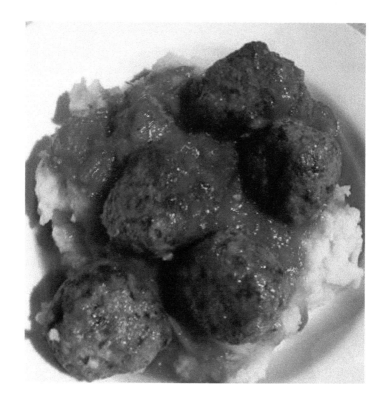

Prep time: 5 mins

Servings: 4

Cooking: 8 mins

Ingredients:

- 400g canned chickpeas
- 4 sprigs of flat parsley
- 4 cup breadcrumbs
- 4 cup olive oil
- 2 cloves garlic
- 2 shallots
- 1 egg

Directions:

1. Peel and chop the shallots and garlic cloves.
2. Rinse and chop the parsley.
3. Rinse and drain the chickpeas.
4. Heat 1 tbsp oil in a nonstick skillet, and fry the garlic and shallots 2 min over medium heat, stirring.
5. Then mix with the chickpeas and parsley and add the egg.
6. Form dumplings with your wet hands, and roll them into the bread crumbs.
7. Heat the remaining oil in a pan and brown the meatballs.
8. Serve with a tomato sauce.

Nutrition:

- Calories 161
- Fat 14.5 g
- Carbs 2 g
- Protein 0.4 g

Lemon Roasted Radishes

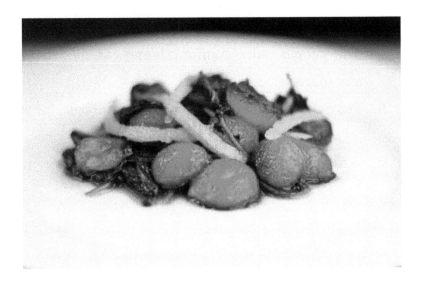

Prep time: 5 mins

Servings: 2

Ingredients:

- 2 bunches rinsed and quartered radishes
- 2 tsps. Lemon juice
- 1½ tsp. roughly fresh chopped rosemary
- 1 tbsp melted coconut oil

Directions:

1. Heat the oven to 350°F. Line a baking sheet with parchment paper.
2. Add pepper, salt, coconut oil, and radishes to a bowl and mix until combined.
3. Place the mixture on a baking sheet and bake for about 35 mins, stirring occasionally.
4. When it is done, toss with rosemary and lemon juice.

Nutrition:

- Calories 37
- Fat 2 g
- Carbs 4 g
- Protein 1 g

Green Beans with Nuts

Prep time: 20 mins

Servings: 2

Ingredients:

- 3 minced garlic cloves
- 1 tbsp olive oil
- ½ cup chopped walnuts
- 2 cup sliced green beans

Directions:

1. Boil the beans in salted water until tender.
2. Place the beans, garlic and walnuts in a preheated pan and cook for about 5-7 mins on the stove.

Nutrition:

- Calories 285
- Fat 24.1 g
- Carbs 7.1 g
- Protein 10 g

Beets Stewed with Apples

Prep time: 1 hour

Servings: 2

Ingredients:

- 2 tbsp Tomato paste
- 1 tbsp Olive oil
- 1 cup water
- 2 peeled, cored and sliced apples
- 3 peeled, boiled and grated beets
- 2 tbsp Sour cream

Directions:

1. Boil the beets until half-done
2. In a deep pan preheated with olive oil cook the grated beets for 15 mins.
3. Add the sliced apples, tomato paste, sour cream and 1 cup water. Stew for 30 mins covered.

Nutrition:

- Calories 346
- Fat 7.7 g
- Carbs 26.8 g
- Protein 2 g

Cabbage Quiche

Prep time: 30 mins

Servings: 4

Cooking: 20 mins

Ingredients:

- 2 beaten eggs
- 2 tbsp Sour cream
- 2 tsps. Semolina
- Fresh parsley
- ½ shredded white cabbage head
- 2 tbsp milk

Directions:

1. In a saucepan stew the shredded cabbage with milk until soft and done.
2. Sprinkle the semolina over the cabbage, constantly stirring, and cook for 10 mins more.

3. Remove from the heat, let cool and stir in the beaten eggs. Season with salt.

4. Arrange the cabbage mixture in a baking dish, coat with sour cream and bake at 400°F for 20 mins.

5. Serve with sour cream and fresh parsley leaves.

Nutrition:

- Calories 93
- Fat 0.5 g
- Carbs 27.8 g
- Protein 19.4 g

Rice and Chicken Stuffed Tomatoes

Prep time: 10 mins

Servings: 4

Cooking: 25 mins

Ingredients:

- 1 pack grilled and sliced chicken breast
- 2 tbsp Chopped basil leaf
- 2 cup cooked brown rice
- 1 tbsp olive oil
- 4 large tomatoes
- ½ cup grated parmesan cheese
- 2 minced garlic cloves

Directions:

1. Set the oven at 350F.
2. Take the top of the tomatoes off and then carefully scoop the seeds using a spoon.

3. In a large bowl, mix together the cooked brown rice, chicken, basil, garlic, and parmesan (leave about 1 tsp. of parmesan). Use this mixture to stuff the tomatoes.
4. Sprinkle the stuffed tomatoes with the remaining parmesan. Place them in an oven-safe dish and brush with the olive oil.
5. Place in the oven to cook for 25 mins.
6. Let it cool down before serving.

Nutrition:

- Calories 230
- Fat 4.1 g
- Carbs 27.3 g
- Protein 21.5 g

Lightning Source UK Ltd.
Milton Keynes UK
UKHW020647100621
385263UK00001B/110